THE MENOPAUSE SOLUTION

Evelyn T. Myers

Without the direct or indirect counsel of a doctor, the author of this book does not provide medical advice or recommend the use of any approach as a form of treatment for physical, emotional, or medical issues. The author's only goal in providing this knowledge is to aid you in your pursuit of mental, physical, and spiritual health. The author and publisher disclaim any liability for your conduct if you utilize any of the information in this book for personal use.

Table of content

Introduction

You can't rewrite history, including your own.

You cannot modify your genetics. You can't change how your life has progressed up to this point, and if you're like most of us, you probably can't change a lot of your current circumstances either. That implies there are some aspects of perimenopause and menopause that you cannot control. But you can change some of it, including simply accepting it and yourself inside it, and you can manage a lot of it.

A great number of studies show that when we enter this phase, even if we are just taught about it and realistically prepared and supported, we will have a better experience. If it hasn't even begun for you, just reading this book will almost certainly make it all better when it does, and I don't say that to impress myself. Even if it has already begun for you, even if it stinks, you can enhance your experience simply by learning more about it.

This is not one of those books in which I, the Great and Powerful Evelyn, discover the mystery of menopause for myself and now can solve it for you so that we can all have a fantastic time and experience and cherish this stage of life as nothing more than a glorious passage of glittering wisdom and wonder.

The concept of me being the master of menopause is particularly amusing, because, let me tell you, I am the dog of menopause. You'll have to go elsewhere for mastery. This is not a comprehensive guide. Everything you need isn't going to be in any book, let alone this one, and even if it was, we both know you wouldn't have half the patience, let alone the stamina, to read its eight thousand pages, let alone haul it up three flights of stairs from the lobby.

Understanding, acceptance, and management of Your Choice are the keywords of the game here:

they are what is genuinely feasible and will not make you feel any worse about yourself than menopause may. As my brilliant friend Anne, a disability activist and writer, pointed out when we discussed this, just like with disability and disabled people, so much historical and current messaging about menopause and those of us in perimenopause or postmenopause treats it and us as broken in need of repair. To be "right" or "balanced," we should try to keep or make ourselves, our hormones, and our bodies as premenopausal as possible, rather than accepting that we, our bodies, and our hormones are always correct, even if we don't always feel comfortable or love every phase of them. This book isn't about how to fix yourself, your hormones, or any other component of your body. I believe you are correct, even though you, like me, are through a particularly difficult period. I'm not here to help you fix yourself. I'm only here to assist you in getting through this hot mess. I believe I can assist you in avoiding becoming stranded in menopause in the first place, or, if that has already occurred, get you through it and aid you. The good news is that even if I can't do either, you probably spent less money on this book than you did on those 10 bottles of herbs or lotions that didn't work.

There is a lot of carefully prescribed Menopause counsel. If someone discovered what worked for them, they would often believe and say that it would fix all of their problems. If someone had anything that didn't work for them or that they couldn't do, they will typically make it the huge, horrible thing that no one should do and may even scare you out of utilizing it although it works very well for you and you have every assurance it's safe for you. Our lives, bodies, and experiences are simply much too diverse for everything or anything to work for (or not work for) all of us or make us feel the same way.

If I or anybody else says anything in here that doesn't square with your experience of your own body and how things have (or haven't) worked or felt for you, I want you to believe yourself, your body, and your expert knowledge of both.

Megan Smith, a nutritional therapy specialist, and community organizer, assisted me with the dietary sections of the book. "Our bodies are complex, with a lot going on inside them," she continues. Most individuals have been socialized in such a way that their ability to listen to that wisdom has been damaged. So much of my work with patients is about restoring that connection and ability to listen. If something doesn't seem right or good, don't do it.

There is no right or wrong way to experience menopause; there is only how we do it.

If you are currently experiencing or will experience difficulties with menopause, whether it is due to physical, mental, emotional, social, or practical effects, or all of the above, it is not because you are a bad or difficult person, lack the proper attitude, or are otherwise doing or have done something wrong. It will primarily be about your genetics, your life and health history, and your current circumstances, all of which you can do little about now and couldn't do much about before. If you're having a good time, it's probably not because of your winning attitude, your weight, or your fitness routine. Of course, things might always change in the future. A challenging one, on the other hand, can.

Whatever the case may be, here's what I believe this book may do for you:

It will explain the current understanding of how perimenopause and menopause occur; what can happen to your body, mind, and life as a result; and why that stuff happens or might happen.

It will provide you with some background information that will make you feel more secure.

It will regale you with tales of my numerous menopausal fascinations and irritants, which you will either enjoy or skip as you get to what you need, and that is entirely up to you, my friend. I will not take it personally.

It will provide you with a plethora of optional considerations for comprehending, digesting, and managing your experience. This is a buffet, not a set menu: you can taste what you want, leave what you don't want, mix it all up, and utilize it however works best for you.

Chapter 1

Menopause In the world of the twenty-first century

We operate under a male way of life. If we decide to have children (19% of us don't), we must take time away from our occupations to have children, and when we return, we must work even harder than our male coworkers to advance in our careers. When we are at the peak of our careers during menopause, we suddenly have to deal with another change in our bodies that men simply don't have to deal with.

When it comes to recognizing menopause, the corporate sector is still so far behind. Although women over 44 have the largest rate of growth in the workforce, 56 percent of those who are going through menopause have had second thoughts about continuing to work, and 11 percent have considered quitting.

We may find ourselves in a boardroom suddenly forgetting what we were about to say, experiencing hot flashes while giving a presentation in front of a large audience, or being entirely worn out from a disturbed night's sleep. Nearly half of the women say they haven't discussed their symptoms with anybody at work, which speaks something about how much of this is handled in silence.

It is quite difficult to go through menopause. Sleepless nights, unstable moods, difficulty losing weight, memory loss, hot flashes, receding hair, dryness in the vagina, and lack of libido are not minor symptoms. Menopause is not like treating a severe virus that only lasts a few weeks. It's a 10-year trip during which our bodies undergo significant change. Symptoms appear to be random and unrelated. They appear and disappear suddenly. You no longer have the hormones that have kept you content, alert, energized, and burning fat.

They are missed. However, they are not returning. We experience this hormonal drop on our own and without enough help, making it a chaotic, crazy, unpredictable ride. I wish to alter that.

Why don't women talk about their menopause journeys more frequently? Why don't we give women more tools for their daily lives to deal with this?

Why aren't women helping one another through this? Menopause is like a high-risk sport. We need a training manual for this adventure. We need to lean in and support one another.

After going through menopause for the past ten years, I realized I wasn't alone. Too many ladies are going through the same thing. Some people have it even worse than others. When women reach this age, they have health issues. It's awful when your hormones begin to fall and your life is flipped upside down. Many of you have contacted me. Your stories have touched me deeply. So much so that it prompted me to pen this book. My health began to deteriorate in my 40s. My 40th birthday was spent in the finest shape of my life. I assumed aging would be a breeze. Nonetheless, my health had deteriorated by the age of 42. My reality became one of hot flashes, insomnia, memory loss, unstable moods, and inexplicable weight gain. I felt like I was living in the body of someone else as if an extraterrestrial had taken over my body. I had lost control of my health. The most difficult aspect of this trip has been that all of my previous techniques for getting my health back on track no longer work.

One of the most difficult aspects of menopause is the complexity of the symptoms. We often don't know when they'll come or how long they'll last, and it's difficult to pinpoint what causes them. For years, many of us have learned to accept our PMS symptoms, which were easy in comparison to the transition into menopause. PMS provides us with a short, hormonal change that just happens right before our periods, and we've found tools to manage them (one of those tools being lots of chocolate). Our relationships can suffer as a result of our mood swings. Anger and irritation are common visitors. Some of us are finding ourselves yelling more at our children and relationships. Even the most insignificant situations might easily provoke us. The most difficult part is that we frequently don't know why. We frequently stroll around annoyed.

I've taught thousands of women through menopause who have told me they've entirely lost their sense of joy in life. It's discouraging when the tiny things that used to make you happy no longer excite you. During these years, many women's memories fade. Too many people find themselves in the middle of a discussion, looking for words and forgetting people's names. A good night's sleep might feel like a luxury for many menopausal women. We are readily roused by any movement or commotion.

Once awake, we spend hours tossing and turning in an attempt to fall back asleep. We wake up soaked in sweat many nights, prompting us to get out of bed to change our clothes and linens. During this time, many of us would do everything to wake up feeling rested.

And then there's the weight gain. Can we briefly discuss the weight gain? It's not right. Do you feel like you're eating the same (or even less), exercising more, and still gaining weight? Menopause comes on suddenly. Too many of us believe we are too young to be experiencing menopause. Menopause was something your mother experienced as she aged.

That isn't you. That cannot be your situation in life.

As challenging as this trip may be for you, I want you to take a minute to stand back from your symptoms and give yourself a fresh perspective. Menopause is an optional experience. It is, in fact, true. The symptoms you are experiencing are your wonderful body's pleas for assistance. You are not required to tolerate them. You are capable of so much more than that. The menopause journey is a wonderful time to tune in and learn what your body needs. Everyone requires something unique. I want to assist you in creating a lifestyle that is tailored to what your body requires.

Symptoms are gifts. I know they don't feel like that while they're happening, but if your body had a language, it would communicate with you through symptoms. Try not to make the process into a villain. Tune in and pay attention. These symptoms manifest for a cause. I understand how difficult it is to live in a body that does not feel like yours. I understand that these symptoms may sap the joy from your life. You've done everything to make yourself feel better, but nothing seems to be working. You've tried numerous herbs, vitamins, drugs, therapies, and diets to feel normal again.

You're at a loss for words and extremely frustrated.

I've got you covered. Assistance is on its way. Consider this book to be a how-to guide for smoothing out the menopausal ride. Your menopausal transition can be an inside-out experience. Instead of looking for something outside of yourself to treat your symptoms, I want to show you how to live a life that supports the changes that are occurring within you, a lifestyle that respects the wisdom that your body possesses. Your external experience will vary as a result. I want to teach you the language of your body and offer you the means to work with it rather than against it.

You will notice that I am a scientific enthusiast. I don't just want to know that something works; I want to know why it works. I developed my entire practice around using healing methods that are not only effective but also have research to back them up. One of the most shocking facts I discovered during my menopause journey was that diseases such as breast cancer, ovarian cancer, heart disease, diabetes, dementia, and Alzheimer's are more common among women in their postmenopausal years. I was curious as to why this was the case. What happens that predisposes women to so many diseases? Our hormones, I realized, are like a symphony. Each instrument contributes to the creation of a lovely piece of music. If one of the instruments breaks, the entire composition will be thrown off. The disease develops as a result of the breakdown of a few hormones. Balancing our hormones when we enter menopause isn't just about retaining our sanity; it's also about saving our lives.

I'm on a mission to help women comprehend this. We can assist a woman in avoiding serious diseases such as cancer, heart disease, dementia, Alzheimer's, and even osteoporosis if we course-correct throughout her menopausal years.

I am honored to be a part of this journey with you. I am a firm believer that everything in our lives happens for a reason. I know my difficulties with menopause occurred so that I could help other ladies going through the same thing.

As you read this book, keep an open mind. Many of the lifestyle strategies I offer are cutting-edge, but they may be the polar opposite of what you have previously been taught. Science informs us otherwise. Today's world is not the same as it was decades ago. As a result, we must approach menopause differently.

I've got some exciting news for you. You can adjust these symptoms no matter where you are in your menopausal journey. And as soon as possible. It does not require a miraculous drug; it can be as simple as making lifestyle adjustments that will work with the hormonal decrease you are experiencing. I'm pleased to share with you the lifestyle skills that have helped me and hundreds of my patients get through this rough patch. I don't believe in miracle cures. I believe in the human body's power. The feminine physique is well-designed. We were designed to carry another human inside of us. Isn't that amazing? This design, however, changes substantially during our menopausal years. There is no magical herb or antidepressant medicine that can remedy that transformation. You must adjust your way of life to accommodate the internal changes.

Power comes from knowledge. The more you understand about your body's processes, the more in control you will feel. Hormones are difficult to comprehend. This book is intended to help you understand and work with your hormones. Hormones are difficult to comprehend. This book is intended to simplify them so that you can work with your hormones rather than against them. You can alleviate your symptoms. You can thrive even throughout menopause. You have more power than you realize. I am thrilled to return that power to you.

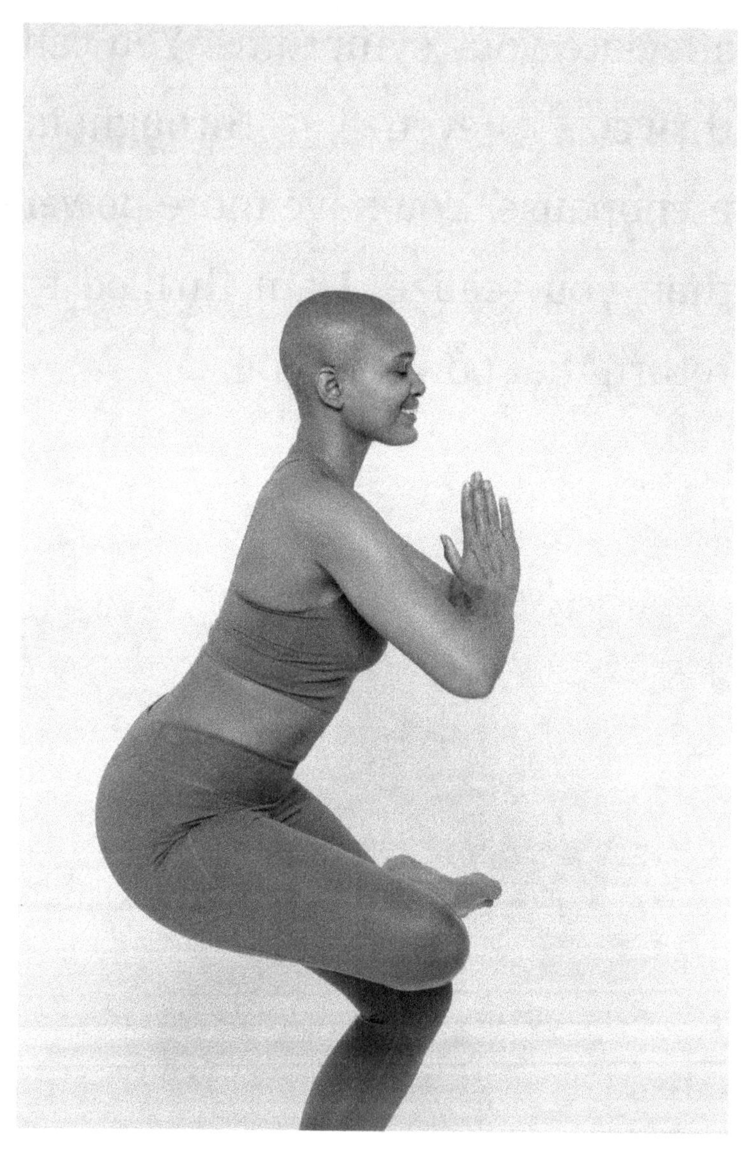

Chapter 2

Welcome to menopause

I'm most likely the least probable person to be writing a book about menopause. I didn't experience many hormonal issues for the majority of my life. My period came and went with no noticeable signs. I never had any issues with my ability to get pregnant. My husband and I decided to try for a baby when I reached 30 and I became pregnant right away. I've never given hormone balancing any thought. Then I turned 40. My hormones led me down a path I never anticipated experiencing. I spent a decade trying to figure out how to get off of that crazy rollercoaster.

Due to my sense of isolation throughout this process, I authored this book.

My symptoms were severe and had a significant impact on my life. However, the only solutions I could find were to put up with the discomfort or take medication. Neither of those choices appealed to me. Since I've been posting about my experience with menopause on social media, I've heard from many of you who have gone through something similar. You too have been severely impacted by menopause. You missed it, just as I did. In my early 40s, I started the menopause process. I transformed from a happy, vivacious, and caring person to an emotional disaster overnight. Sincerely, I had the impression that someone had taken control of my thoughts, sleep, and general well-being. My life and relationships were disrupted, and I eventually stopped loving the person I had become. It also served as the impetus for a search that lasted ten years and enabled me to end my hormonal lunacy as well as turn around and assist thousands of women who are navigating the ups and downs of menopause.

I wanted to be in the best form of my life when I turned 40. At that time in my life, that meant reaching a specific weight on the bathroom scale or fitting into my favorite pair of skinny pants. I believe that maintaining good health requires a balanced diet and regular exercise. My standard of health was based on external observations. I reasoned that if I thought I looked well on the outside, I must be in good health on the inside. My 40th birthday passed by without any notice. I had heard complaints about how difficult it was to lose weight from other women who had reached the age of 40. I didn't go through that. I had the impression that I was unstoppable. My life was perfect at the time. I had a wonderful spouse, two wonderful children, ages 10 and 8 at the time, flourishing health practices, and a fantastic group of friends. Soon after turning 40, I started going through severe depressive waves. It came on suddenly, made me cry for no apparent reason, and left me feeling helpless.

The waves started modest and irregular, but as my 40s went on, they started happening more frequently. It took me some time to realize how depressed I had become. I kept trying to rediscover my delight by utilizing all of my mental strategies, but nothing was working.

Nothing about this made sense. There was nothing in my life that I could point to and say, "That's it," such as a trigger or traumatic experience. That's why I'm feeling so down.

Those years of despair taught me that there will always be things in life that make us sad. When things don't go as we had hoped, depression results. I suffered that kind of depression up until I was in my early forties. But this seemed unique. It was simply deep and irrational, which is all I could say to characterize it. On paper, my life was the American dream, but I wanted to leave it behind. To those of you who have previously experienced this type of depression, my heart goes out to you. Hard going. It appeared as though something had seized possession of my thoughts and I was no longer in charge.

I had a lot of knowledge about physical health at this time in my professional career but little knowledge of mental health. I started researching other techniques, including yoga, meditation, chiropractic adjustments, and acupuncture. I sought advice from people who had already experienced depression as well as from inspirational authors and lecturers. These tools were all helpful, but only momentarily.

Panic attacks immediately followed depression waves. Anxiety began to appear frequently. At night, I would awaken with an overwhelming sense of dread. I would perform what I called my worry scan a lot of the time. I would be startled out of a deep slumber when two in the morning would arrive. Anxiety, fear, and panic would rule. To make sense of this panic, my mind tried to give it a cause. I would immediately go over every area of my life where anything had gone wrong. I would toss and turn for the next two hours, trying to reason through issues that, in some cases, weren't even there. I couldn't stop it, and it seemed like madness. The nightly heat flashes then started. I would have to change clothing several times in a single night because they were so awful. I would need to wake up my husband to change my wet sheets since they were that bad. To avoid waking him up, I began to sleep in a sleeping bag in our bed. The anxiety and heat flushes made it difficult to fall asleep. It would be simple to conclude that this marked the traditional onset of menopause, but I was only 43 years old and had a regular cycle. The menopause typically begins at age 55.

This truly was awful. I had not anticipated my health in my 40s to look like this. I was aware that my body was experiencing hormonal issues, but I was unable to identify the root of the problem.

What practical resource was I missing? What was more essential was how I was going to get out of this.

I have never been hesitant to seek assistance when I need it. Fortunately, I was surrounded by a wonderful group of knowledgeable women. I began by contacting my older sister. She acknowledged that she had some anxiety and sadness when she was my age and had found medications to be a helpful treatment. What is her suggestion? Perhaps it was time to consider using medication. It was seductive. This nightmare would end if you took a medication. I hadn't taken any pharmaceuticals in years, and as a holistic physician, I was aware that doing so would merely provide a band-aid solution and not address the underlying problem. I was also aware of research on the long-term health effects of persistent antidepressant use. The difficulty of stopping antidepressant use after starting them is possibly their largest drawback. I didn't want to drastically alter my neurochemical system. I didn't want to spend the rest of my life depending on medicine to make me happy. There had to be a different approach. I had to have a good cause for feeling this way. I made contact with my friends, many of whom were between five and ten years older than me. They told me to "buck up" in response. Your perimenopause is starting. It's going to be a rough ride, so prepare yourself. 43 years of age? It was still illogical. Years ago, my mother used to talk about how simple menopause was for her. In her early 50s, she passed through menopause without a hot flash or gloomy moment in sight. I was without a doubt lacking something.

One evening, I was at my child's school science fair and happened to be standing next to one of the mothers, an OB/GYN who was well-known in our neighborhood. I approached her and explained my predicament because I was in a desperate state and had run out of options. She responded to me in a way that fundamentally altered how I would always view health.

I wish I had an answer for you, Evelyn, she added. I have a lot of women your age in my practice who are experiencing those hormonal symptoms, and I genuinely don't know how to treat them.

The medical texts I have are useless to me. I did not anticipate that response. For weeks after our chat, the phrases "my medical textbooks have failed me" and "a practice full of women who have those hormonal symptoms" kept playing in my head. There has to be an environmental component to this hormonal condition if it affects so many women. Everything for me changed that evening. It catalyzed me to learn how to reset hundreds of women's menopause symptoms using the same strategies I did. It took me years of study and perseverance to comprehend and use these skills, but they are what restored my life, and they will do the same for you.

My desire to learn why this was occurring to so many women and what I could do to resolve my health crisis was stoked by our chat that evening. It led me down a path of fascinating research that demonstrates that there is an epidemic of anxiety, depression, and thyroid issues among women today.

The medical literature has failed us, to be sure.

I have devoted the last ten years to learning about how the poisonous environment of today affects women. I have also become fixated on all the scientific evidence showing us how adept our bodies are at self-detoxifying through the use of methods like fasting and the ketogenic diet. I can genuinely say that, as I sit here in my fifties, I am a happier, healthier, and more energetic version of the person I was when I was forty. I was able to regain my joy and sanity using the methods I've provided in this book. I have no trouble falling asleep and staying asleep all night. Night sweats are an uncommon guest. Depression is unable to penetrate my head. When an anxiety attack does occasionally creep up on me, I am ready and have the resources to quickly recover. I experience strength and control. I sense myself once more.

My experience with menopause gave me a strong urge to show women how to approach this stage of life in a new way. We don't need to endure pain. We do not need to create sickness. Menopause can be a chance for us to start over with our health and be our best for years to come. I consistently witness these measures helping women. I created my clinic around the idea of giving menopausal women the chance to reset their health since I have grown so enthusiastic about it. I built programs that unite women in a setting of mutual support and provide them with skills to deal with their symptoms. Finally, I developed a detoxification program that is specially designed to get rid of the chemicals that damage women's hormones.

Never stop believing in yourself. You were given the most incredible, self-healing body at birth. All you have to do is discover how to activate the healing process. I'm eager to travel with you on this adventure. You merit to lead a joyful life.

This book is a summary of my research and the steps I took to improve the health of the women in my practice and online community as well as my own.

It is a gift I'm giving you. I sincerely hope you discover the solutions you've been looking for here.

Chapter 3

Time to begin paying attention to your body

You must pause and pay attention to how your body is changing. How frequently do you ignore your body's signals? Since the beginning of our periods, we've learned to keep premenstrual syndrome (PMS) and all other emotions we experience during our cycles internalized. However, I believe that this is beginning to change for our daughters, just as the conversation around menopause is beginning to change as well. In my practice, I frequently work with kids, and I'm constantly amazed by how they instinctively pay attention to their bodies. Sadly, as adults, we've outgrown this behavior. We internalize a lot of the stress that comes from society, including racism and sexism, as well as from attempting to balance having a family and/or work. At perimenopause, we have to recognize that we can no longer maintain the level of physical and emotional activity we did in our twenties and thirties. When we start to shift our boundaries or say no to people, we start to ruffle their feathers. shift is sometimes a difficult process for those around us. However, I believe that in the long run, everyone benefits because when we change behavior patterns that aren't serving us well, we feel happier and more content.

Symptom Reset for Menopause
Whatever stage of menopause you are in, I want to show you how to reset your symptoms. The chapters that follow contain some fantastic tools that can help you alter the course of your health. The purpose of this book, which I set out to write, was to instruct women on how to relieve their menopause symptoms. The hero of the day isn't your doctor, your

friends' quick-fix diet, or a magic pill that will cure all of your symptoms. You are the hero. You have magic in you.

Your body was built to heal itself. There is a way of living that will accelerate that mending. However, it is not as easy as simply going for a jog or performing a single three-day water fast. To survive during these years, you will need to implement several lifestyle adjustments.

The ketotic diet, eating to regulate your hormones, detoxing to get rid of poisonous estrogens, and mindfulness exercises may all be in your toolbox. As a holistic physician for many years, I've noticed that when individuals initially decide to attempt a more alternative, natural approach to treatment, they bring the perspective that mainstream medicine teaches with them. the philosophy of "one pill, one diagnosis."

Consider the blood pressure. Your blood pressure is elevated when you enter the doctor's office. What is your doctor going to do? Give you a prognosis and a prescription most likely, right? Say you decide against taking the drug. A more organic strategy is what you want. You start looking for that one thing that can naturally lower your blood pressure. What if your blood pressure increased for no apparent reason? What if the causes were numerous? The answer is beyond a single natural supplement.

You'll discover that with your menopause symptoms.

Most likely, multiple factors are contributing to your symptoms. There are probably multiple contributing factors. Don't let this get you down. I've created a list of five significant lifestyle adjustments you can make to start feeling better. To name a few, they're altering when and what you eat, nourishing your microbiota, reducing your toxic load, and managing your stress. I'll start by explaining how your body functions. I'll then give you tips on how to work with your body to improve its performance. I'll finish by providing methods you can follow to master the principles. I'll outline how to put it all together at the end of this book and provide resources to help you on your menopause reset journey. Never give up no matter what. I placed those steps there on purpose. When you are overloaded with information, it is simple for limiting beliefs to surface. You may hear gibberish in your head, such as "This is way too hard," "I could never do this," or "What will my friends and family think of me?" Don't pay attention to those ideas. I deliver my lessons by how your body would like you to care for it. When you work with your body's design, changing your lifestyle will feel natural. I frequently witness this. When we improve someone's gut flora, their insatiable sweet tooth disappears. Someone will confess to me that nothing will ever be able to satisfy their sweet tooth. All we had to do was alter the body's blueprint, and the symptoms disappeared.

The five lifestyle modifications that make up your menopause solution are listed below.

Adjust the Time You Eat and What You Eat
Make Your Microbiome Better
Cleanse Your Life and Yourself
Stop Hurrying

A step can be built upon another. Take it one step at a time, much like climbing a steep staircase. Before you know it, all the pieces of a lovely lifestyle that works for you will be in place.

That is what took place with Martha. She was in the menopause at the age of 49. Her new normal included night sweats, anxiety, memory loss, hair loss, chronic fatigue, increasing cholesterol levels, and unexplained weight gain. She was accustomed to working out her way through any symptom because she was a successful athlete. Exercise was not the solution for the first time in her life. The more she exercised, the worse her symptoms were. Martha was the type of person who ate six meals a day and loaded up on carbohydrates when I first started working with her. She had been up with the attitude that breakfast was the most significant meal of the day.

For Martha, the menopausal solution lifestyle was completely novel. Many of the things I suggested to her seemed to go against everything she had ever learned about health. But her tried-and-true methods failed.

She was aware that a change was necessary. She immediately started taking the actions I had just described. I began by pushing back Martha's breakfast by an hour. This presented a challenge for her at first. But she soon got the hang of it, and after a few weeks, she was intermittently fasting every day. She had more energy just from taking this first step. I then needed to get Martha off of a diet that was strong in carbohydrates. She began by cutting out foods high in refined carbs, such as bread and pasta. She was able to extend her fast because this reduced her appetite. She lost the abdominal fat that had gathered over the previous few years as her fast lasted longer. She had more energy, felt less hungry, and was losing weight, so I checked her gut to determine what kind of beneficial bacteria she was harboring. It was discovered that she had a severe lack of beneficial microorganisms that lower cholesterol, break down estrogen that is poisonous, and boost metabolism. She started to include more foods high in polyphenols, probiotics, and prebiotics in her diet. I observed a decrease in her cholesterol after taking this step, as well as alterations to her skin and hair.

Her hazardous burden needed to be reduced as a final stage. According to Martha's heavy metal test, she had abnormally high lead and mercury levels. I showed her how to open up her detox pathways first, and then eliminate toxins from her body and brain.

This method allowed her to get rid of those poisons safely and successfully. Martha regained her life at the final step.

Her anxiety subsided, her hair stopped falling out, and night sweats ceased occurring as she began to sleep through the night.

Even though Martha wasn't yet in menopause, she now had the means to minimize her symptoms.

After completing the preceding steps, Martha examined her hectic schedule. She added downtime, declined more invites that would tire her, and we even convinced her to mix up her exercise routine more. With each step, Martha learned a new way of life. At first, each step seemed alien. But as she persisted, each step became simpler and more comfortable. The wonderful aspect is that she returned to each step at a higher level of health. Martha recently underwent a hormone test, and the results were fantastic and beautifully balanced.

She was ready to go through menopause with little symptoms and no risk of illness.

You can follow Martha's example. She possessed no special abilities beyond what you already possess. Assemble the steps. Recognize that this technique consistently produces positive results.

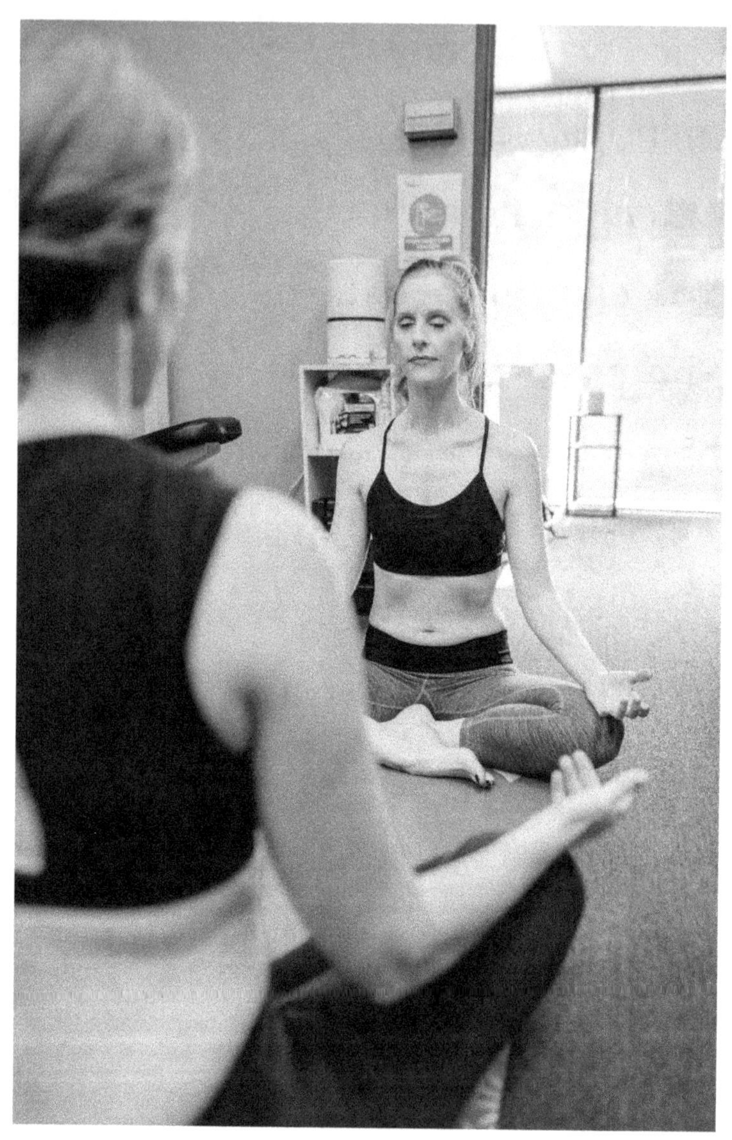

Chapter 4

Increases and decreases in hormone levels

I desire for you to control your hormones. This necessitates having a fundamental understanding of which hormones will affect you the most during menopause. Additionally, you should become familiar with the bodily organs that generate these hormones. Your endocrine system is composed of these organs. I'll introduce you to the endocrine systems in this chapter that have the biggest impact on your symptoms. I'll also discuss some of my go-to methods for figuring out your hormonal profile and which hormones need the most attention.

Let's return to the structure of your body. Whether you like it or not, a large part of your design as a woman is focused on preparing for and giving birth to a child. Your body and mind have been impacted neurochemically by hormones that have a significant impact on how you feel ever since you entered puberty. You would be amazed at how many neurochemicals have to collaborate each month to bring you happiness, aid in sleep, calm you, make you look beautiful, maintain full hair and wrinkle-free skin, lubricate your mucous membranes, increase your sex drive, enable multitasking, inspire you to exercise, and even give you the gift of gab. You have experienced a magnificent symphony of hormones that have aided you in a variety of ways since you first entered puberty. The absence of all those beneficial hormones is a challenge for menopausal women.

This hormonal decrease starts in your forties, but it doesn't happen gradually or consistently. They become crazy. There are days when they are higher than usual and days when they are nonexistent. This is what sends your emotions into a tailspin and gives you the impression that something is seriously wrong with you. From a hormonal standpoint, you can have the hormones of an adolescent one day and be utterly hormone-depleted the next day, similar to a postmenopausal lady. This roller coaster ride was bumpy for me. My emotional highs and lows were so strong that I was never sure if I would be overcome with appreciation and joy or if I would want to kill anyone who mistreated me.

Although I detested it, the wild ups and downs gave me the ability to understand my body better.

You will discover that there are many social misconceptions about how the female hormonal system functions as you go deeper into studying hormones. For instance, did you know that multiple organs in your body regulate your hormones? They are managed by a collection of organs. This mistake frequently occurs with thyroid disorders. It's typical for women to visit their doctor when their metabolism starts acting up, and the doctor will check their thyroid to make sure it's functioning normally. But that organ doesn't function by itself. Her brain's pituitary and hypothalamus must guide it. A thyroid disease can never be entirely cured by treating the thyroid as an independent organ. You must speak to the entire team.

Your hormones are produced by endocrine glands, which are organs. Every endocrine organ functions as a team. Even their names are unique to these teams. For instance, you might be familiar with the HPA axis as one of the teams. This group of endocrine glands, which also comprises your pituitary and hypothalamus as well as your adrenal glands, is known as your adrenal team. To give you energy and mental clarity under stressful situations, this team creates cortisol. Your sex hormone team, known as the HPO axis, has also been working very hard for you. Your ovaries serve as the endocrine gland, and your pituitary and hypothalamus are also members of this team. All testosterone, progesterone, and estrogen production is managed by your HPO axis team.

The HPO axis crew starts to slow down as soon as you turn forty. It has been doing its job for about thirty years, and now it is no longer motivated to work.

The HPO axis must delegate its responsibility to another team because your body still requires some sex hormones. The HPA axis is the group it gives it to. The menopausal lunacy starts at this handoff.

Due to the physical, mental, and chemical stress many of you have been experiencing, your HPA axis team has been working extra hard for years. Your sex hormones will swiftly drop off after your HPO axis crew leaves and the HPA axis team takes control. You'll experience a drop in mood, anxiety, insomnia, sex drive, muscle loss, weight gain, and a sense of insanity as a result of this deterioration. This is precisely what occurred to me. The difficult aspect is figuring out who in the team is having trouble and needs assistance. Chasing your falling hormones with herbs or pharmaceuticals will frequently leave you disappointed and without solutions because there are so many players in the hormonal game. You can improve your health beyond anything you've ever known if you're prepared to put in the effort to learn about your body and everything that goes into creating your hormonal picture. After menopause, the majority of hormonal malignancies, like breast and ovarian cancer, develop. We may spare women in their postmenopausal years a great deal of hardship if doctors could help them learn how to manage their hormones as they go through the menopause years. It's important to go through this phase of menopause. Your body will start to show all of its imbalances. It can be lifesaving to recognize these imbalances and make the decision to correct them. The menopause is a fantastic opportunity to start over with your health. In our younger years, we focused a lot on starting families, establishing careers, and taking care of our neighbors. We have a chance to take care of ourselves throughout the menopause years. To be at our best in our latter years, we should want to take insane care of our health.

During these years, adjusting your hormones can seem like a

daunting task. At times, it may seem alluring to take a pill to address your issues. You will not only alleviate your problems today if you persevere and pay attention to your body, but your future self will also appreciate you. I tell them to be patient and to prepare a toolkit as we piece together their hormonal picture. There will still be highs and lows as you go through these years. That cannot be avoided. However, you can decide how low the lows go. Making a specialized toolset for menopausal ladies is what I have found to be most beneficial. Each person's toolkit will be unique. For many of you, for instance, removing heavy metals from your hypothalamus and pituitary will balance your melatonin levels and help you sleep again, while for others, overcoming insulin resistance requires reducing your carbohydrate intake and learning how to live a fasting lifestyle.

Knowing which tool can balance which hormone becomes quite beneficial because menopause is a process. It returns you to the driver's seat.

Be Willing to Prioritize Yourself

I'm aware that you've been giving your all to those around you, but right now, it's time to invest your heart and soul into yourself. Hormone decline indicates decreased protection. During the menopausal transition, you are more susceptible to illness than before.

There are some of the best methods for resetting your hormones in this book, but prioritizing yourself is the only thing that will truly save your life. The years leading up to menopause will show you where your imbalances are unlike any other time in your life. It will catch up to you if you have been leading an overscheduled, hectic life. As your hormones deteriorate, you may no longer be able to eat whatever you want without experiencing negative consequences. Your way of life might require an extreme overhaul if you wish to prosper throughout these years. However, it all begins with taking a deep breath and putting yourself first right away.

Avoid assuming; test

This is the moment when testing is most important because there are so many participants in your hormonal picture. The DUTCH Complete Hormone Test is the test that I value the most. I adore this test since it is simple to administer and provides a comprehensive picture of all the hormones involved in a menopausal woman's experience.

The urine test for the DUTCH is done at home. On the website of my practice, you can order this test. Five different urine samples are collected for the test throughout 12 hours. Your sex hormones—estrogen, progesterone, and testosterone—will be examined, and the results will reveal exactly what is happening. Additionally, it provides a reading for the health of your adrenals. Determining whether your adrenal glands are releasing enough cortisol at the appropriate time of day, is incredibly beneficial. It may help you gain a better knowledge of your happy-making chemicals, such as serotonin and dopamine.

This accurate test will also indicate how well you are methylating or how well your body is eliminating pollutants. You may even check to see how much melatonin your pineal gland is producing. Can you see why I enjoy taking this exam? It's very thorough and comprehensive.

The DUTCH test's breakdown of your estrogen metabolites may be what I appreciate the best. A fancy phrase used to describe what transpires to a chemical after it has been broken down is called "metabolites." In this instance, an estrogen metabolite is a crucial indicator of the breakdown of your total estrogen. Sometimes the metabolization of hormones results in disease-causing metabolites. With estrogen, this is particularly accurate. A woman may avert a lot of hormonal malignancies if she knows what her estrogen is decomposing into.

There are three distinct estrogen metabolites in you. One is protective and will aid in lowering the risk of cardiovascular disease and hormonal malignancies. Two are dangerous and will result in numerous malignancies. Knowing your balance of these estrogens is essential for maintaining good health both now and in the future. You can use detox procedures to increase the protective estrogen and decrease the dangerous estrogens once you are aware of your estrogen metabolite balance.

I'll be open and honest with you. I never gave my hormones much thought before beginning my menopause adventure. I never acknowledged the happiness they brought me or the positive effects they had on my health. I delved into learning about progesterone when the waves of anxiety first began to wash over me. I had no idea that this wonderful hormone appeared to me once a month to soothe me and relax my body. She left after that, and I would do anything to get her back. When I was driving to work on an anxious day, I wondered, "Did I ever take progesterone for granted? That hormone was such a blessing to me.

Since then, I've discovered that many women are unaware of how their hormones affect their well-being. You will benefit from knowing what these hormones do as menopause is the time when they are increasing and decreasing.

I frequently advise my clients that they should have a fundamental understanding of the hormones involved in their menopause journey if they wish to balance their hormones and feel like themselves again. I actually behaved in this way when my hormones became out of control. I went back to my textbooks and did a thorough study of the beginning of the chapter on female physiology. Since knowledge is power, I felt helpless. I want to return that power to you throughout the following few pages.

Hormones are a moving target. As you walk through menopause, you never know which hormones may arrive or go. The first step to recovering a sense of control is to learn which hormones cause which symptoms. Knowing the basics about your hormones will help you decide which techniques to employ at what time.

Your hormonal hierarchy comes first. Do you realize that not all hormones are created equally? Some hormones are more powerful than others. Most likely, when you think about menopause, you associate the symptoms with the three sex hormones estrogen, progesterone, and testosterone. You might wish to bring up these hormones when they start to decline, which would seem to make sense. However, three additional hormones have a significant impact on your sex hormones. If you don't maintain a healthy balance of these three hormones, you'll fight the natural drop of your sex hormones and never feel like yourself again.

The enjoyable part is now here. Guess which hormone dominates the hierarchy? Oxytocin. Keep this hormone in mind. The moment you hold your child for the first time if you are a mother, this hormone rushes through you. Recall how amazing that felt. Ever experienced love? Guess what, every time you saw your loved one, oxytocin gave you that amazing, delicious feeling inside of you. Is anyone here a fan of animals? The hormone oxytocin is responsible for our feelings of calm and relaxation when we cuddle with our pets.

The most effective hormone is oxytocin.

The fact that our hormonal system is at the top of the hormone food chain is a lovely feature of its design. You make great strides towards regulating your sex hormones when you experience a lot of oxytocin rushing through you. How fantastic is that?

Cortisol is the following hormone in line. I am aware of that. That awful cortisol. This is the one that consistently throws your health off balance. Cortisol causes you to gain unwanted belly fat, spikes your blood sugar, and wakes you up at two in the morning to let you know there is a crisis. Your body releases a large amount of cortisol whenever you experience or think you are experiencing stress. Cortisol will even manifest itself if you have a packed agenda of enjoyable activities. The rushing woman's hormone is cortisol.

Your sex hormones are greatly affected by this hormone. Lowering your cortisol surges is essential, as I have dealt with thousands of women going through the menopausal transition. If you don't get your cortisol under control, it will be difficult for you to lose weight, have a decent night's sleep, or feel comfortable in your skin.

Insulin is positioned underneath cortisol. This hormone helps you lose weight. When you eat, your pancreas releases insulin. More insulin is released when a meal contains more sugar. You will continue to release insulin if you continue eating a high-sugar, high-carb diet. If the insulin you get through diet is more than your body can handle, it will be stored as fat. Before you force your body to access that fat, it may be sitting there for years. It won't be enough to just start changing your diet if you struggle to lose weight during menopause, which is why I have all my patients going through menopause adopt a fasting lifestyle. Now we come to your sex hormones, which are at the bottom of the hierarchy because they can be significantly influenced by the hormones above. You have three sex hormones. Our culture blames estrogen for diseases like breast cancer or for making us more sensitive to emotional pain. However, not all estrogen is bad. In many respects, it does benefit us.

Around day twelve of your cycle, estrogen has been increasing in your body for most of your life. Your ovaries receive this surge as a signal to release an egg that is ready for implantation. If you have children, estrogen likely played a significant role in making sure you had a ready-made egg. You couldn't become pregnant if your estrogen levels weren't right. Oestrogen also makes you look beautiful. Let's return to your ingenious creation. Your body is prepared to give birth when estrogen levels rise and an egg is released. Oestrogen will make you as beautiful as possible to make sure you mate. To make you appear child-ready, this entails thickening your hair, giving you smooth, plump skin, and even packing some additional fat into your hips. Yes, believe it or not, there is a ratio between our waist and our hips that is said to enhance our attractiveness. Once again for reproductive purposes, estrogen helps to keep your vaginal membranes well-lubricated.

Having said all of that, you should be aware that estrogen has a negative side. We have three different kinds of estrogens (metabolites), two of which are harmful and one of which is beneficial. You put yourself at risk of getting hormonal cancers like breast and ovarian if you let the harmful ones grow and don't feed the protective ones.

Progesterone is the next sex hormone and has been your friend for years. It wasn't until it started to go that I realized how amazing this sex hormone was. As I entered my "menopause years," my progesterone levels dropped, which left me with irregular cycles, anxiety, and a lack of relaxation in my skin.

On day twenty-one of your cycle, progesterone has abundantly entered your life. It was the cause of your uterus's monthly bleeding and shedding. You're calmed by progesterone. It also prevents estrogen from misbehaving. Progesterone and estrogen interact oppositely. Oestrogen might become out of control if progesterone levels drop. A variety of menopause symptoms must be managed by maintaining this estrogen/progesterone balance.

For women going through menopause, low progesterone frequently presents problems. When you begin to bleed days before your period, you have low progesterone. Or perhaps you've had exceptionally heavy periods that make you feel like you're bleeding. Because of the stress demands they had in their thirties and forties, progesterone levels in women experience low points throughout menopause. Why does progesterone drop so dramatically as you approach menopause?

Many women experience low levels of progesterone as a result of low levels of the steroid hormone DHEA. Progesterone, testosterone, and cortisol are produced by the body using DHEA through a sequence of chemical processes. Your body will always put stress first, so if you've been stressed out for a long time, your DHEA reserves may have been diverted to the production of cortisol. You can become low on both progesterone and testosterone as a result. This is where a thorough hormone test, like the DUTCH test, might be useful in determining your precise DHEA levels. Increased DHEA levels can aid in the production of more progesterone. And finally, testosterone. Although testosterone is often associated with men, women can also greatly benefit from this hormone. You benefit from testosterone most in three key areas: sex, drive, and muscle development. Your sex urge is caused by testosterone. Additionally, it is what inspires you to pursue your goals or find the urge to work out. You'll be able to maintain muscle mass more easily as you age if your body has high levels of testosterone. Your menopause symptoms may be significantly impacted by low testosterone. Low sex drive, no desire to exercise, and observable muscle loss are some of the common signs I find in menopausal women. It's a problem with testosterone.

Now that you are aware of the primary hormones involved in

your menopausal experience, let's look at how this hormonal hierarchy functions. Cortisol levels rise when stress levels do. Your blood sugar increases along with cortisol levels. Insulin will increase as blood sugar levels rise. At this time, your body starts storing fat more quickly than usual. Insomnia, hair loss, anxiety, hot flashes, brain fog, resistance to weight reduction, low sex drive, vaginal dryness, and muscle loss are just a few of the symptoms that can result from high levels of cortisol and insulin, which start to accelerate the fall of your sex hormones. Sounds recognizable?

Adjusting Insulin

Balancing insulin is one of the first techniques I employ with my patients. Unbelievably, balancing this hormone may be the simplest. Every time you eat and every time you fast, you have power over your insulin levels. When you learn when and what to consume, resetting your insulin levels becomes a fairly easy chore. I'll demonstrate in this chapter how to adjust the timing of your meals to regulate your insulin levels. Let's look back at your ancestors' prehistoric lifestyles to have a better understanding of how insulin functions in your body. Your body's design has mostly remained unchanged since the days of the cavewoman, although we now live in a modern age with significant technical advancements. Women who lived in caves at that time didn't always have access to food. They lacked refrigeration. They would frequently go days without access to food throughout the winter. Your body is already set up to survive without food. The cavewoman would typically wake up without any food and would have to wait until it was hunted or gathered before she could eat. She wouldn't have breakfast and her blood sugar would fall. Her insulin levels decreased as her blood sugar levels did. But she was unaffected by this. Ketones, an alternative fuel, were used in the construction of her. Her liver would begin producing ketones when her insulin and blood sugar levels were low enough. Her brain was affected by ketones, which increased her alertness, gave her energy, and reduced joint inflammation. Everything she did was done to enable her to go get food.

Let's fast-forward to the present. For our meals, we don't need to go hunting. Breakfast is regarded as the most significant meal of the day, as taught to us. We've all heard that your metabolism increases in speed as you eat more food. Nothing is more false than it is. You have the same design that the cavewoman had thousands of years ago. Like your cavewoman ancestors, you were created for what we call feast/famine cycling. Contravening this design has led to an all-day release of insulin in several women. Your pancreas receives a signal every time you eat to produce insulin. The fastest way to develop insulin is to eat continuously. Your pancreas continues to produce insulin, and as a result, your cells gradually develop a resistance to the insulin that is being delivered to them. Changing how frequently you eat is the first step in controlling your insulin levels. It's simpler than you would imagine. Before doing anything else when I first sit down with a patient, I focus on the timing of her meals. She currently eats throughout the day with constant insulin spikes; I want to switch her to a feast/famine cycle.

This is more in line with the way her body was intended to function. Here is the mindset I want you to have if you are new to feast-and-famine cycling. You should have a window of time where you fast and a window of time where you eat every twenty-four hours. You may have just fasted when you slept up until this point. You might only go six to eight hours without eating after that. This is not enough time to allow your insulin levels to decrease. It's not long enough to induce your body to generate ketones or to reverse insulin resistance. You should strive to practice intermittent fasting, as I request of you. Thirteen to fifteen hours without eating is the first type of intermittent fasting I want you to master. Seem like a difficult task? I'll show you a quick route there.

Simply delaying your breakfast by an hour is the simplest first step towards intermittent fasting. This initial step can be difficult for many of the women I work with.

When you initially make this shift, you could feel queasy, hungry, and a little irritable. But keep in mind that you've educated your body to anticipate breakfast. This exercise has conflicted with the structure of your body. Going against your basic design can have a significant impact on your mood, the amount of fat you store, and the amount of sex hormones you produce. When you treat your body the way it was intended to be treated, you'll be amazed at how rapidly it heals.

I want you to practice moving breakfast back two hours once you've mastered moving it back an hour. Spend a few weeks with it until it starts to feel easy. Continue delaying your meals as the fasting process progresses to the point where you feel comfortable lasting each day for 15 hours without eating.

Adopting an intermittent fasting lifestyle can:

Defy aging by going slowly

Boost your memory.

Insulin resistance can be overcome

Support your weight loss

Defend you against neurological conditions including Alzheimer's and dementia

 Avoid cancer.

decrease arthritis

reverse the effects of asthma

halt the spread of autoimmune diseases

lengthen your life

How to Develop a Fasting Lifestyle

1. Delay breakfast by one hour.

2. Continue delaying breakfast until you feel confident going fifteen hours.

3. Incorporate intermittent fasting (13 to 15 hours without food) into your everyday regimen.

4. Follow a dinner-to-dinner fast on one day per week.

5. When you have mastered the aforementioned stages, you can begin experimenting with various fasts.

Your body can heal itself through fasting in so many amazing ways. I urge you to read my book on dieting for middle-aged women if you are new to fasting and are unsure.

Chapter 5

Ketogenic treatments for menopause

After discussing when to eat, let's go on to discussing what to eat. I want to explain to you in this chapter what foods you can eat to assist in increasing these dwindling hormones. If you are like many women, you have probably spent a lot of your life trying to lose weight. You reduced your calorie intake and increased your workout when you wanted to lose weight. One of the worst methods for reducing weight is what we call the "calories-in, calories-out" approach. Just consider the obesity pandemic we are currently seeing. So many women are starving themselves by consuming only chemical-filled, low-fat diets and trying to burn off those foods by working out for lengthy periods. This method of weight loss is not only challenging to maintain but can also interfere with your metabolism and make future weight loss more difficult. I'm telling you to quit tracking calories, not to stop exercising.

What do you count if you don't count calories? Keep in mind that the goal of this book is to teach you how to use your lifestyle to balance your hormones. Your calorie intake won't always help with your hormones' rollercoaster journey. You can control your diet by what you consume.

I want you to start thinking about your meals in terms of macronutrients from now on. The macronutrients that contribute to your food's calorie content are referred to as macros. Carbohydrates, protein, and fat are the three macronutrients I want you to pay attention to. Each of these macros will have a specific function for you as you go through menopause. Your insulin levels will be raised differently by each.

Recall the hierarchy of hormones. Sex hormones are influenced by insulin. Making sure your diet isn't regularly raising your insulin levels is the first step in starting the process of balancing estrogen, progesterone, and testosterone. Examining the yearly blood tests your doctor performs for you is a wonderful place to start if you want to understand how your food impacts your insulin levels. Your doctor will typically perform a full blood study when you visit for your annual checkup. Hemoglobin

A1C is a measurement that is included in this blood test. Your three-month trend in your insulin levels is revealed by your hemoglobin A1C. For longevity and disease prevention, you want that number to be under three.

Using a home blood sugar reader, which you can readily acquire at your neighborhood drugstore, to regularly monitor your blood sugar levels will help you determine how much insulin your body may be making. Insulin levels will rise in response to a rise in blood sugar. Using an at-home reader is the most effective technique I've found to gauge your blood sugar levels. I advise all of my patients to check their blood sugar in the morning. On most days, you want milligrams per deciliter (mg/DLS) measurement to be between 70 and 90. If it is persistently higher than that, you might be pressuring your pancreas to produce an excessive amount of insulin, which would disrupt your entire hormonal cascade.

How can nutrition help you maintain healthy blood sugar and insulin levels? Your macros are the key, ultimately. To help you comprehend each of these macros, let's dissect it.

Carbohydrates

Carbohydrates are the macronutrient that normally causes the most rise in insulin and blood sugar levels. The largest effect on insulin will be caused by refined carbs, such as those found in breads, pasta, and sweets. Your blood sugar will increase less and your insulin levels won't rise as much if you consume fibrous carbs like those found in fruits and vegetables.

Eliminating refined carbs from your diet is one of the first steps in managing elevated insulin levels. This one alteration, similar to intermittent fasting, might significantly lessen your "menopause symptoms." You might notice an immediate increase in energy, a decrease in appetite, and an improvement in mental clarity if you combine intermittent fasting with a diet low in refined carbohydrates. With my patients, I frequently witness this happening. Following completion of this step, you should begin counting your macros. I advise using an app to keep track of your macros while you get used to the idea of counting macros. There are several excellent apps available to assist you in doing this.

Get a carb manager app and start recording your meals every day.

You want to keep your net carbs under fifty grams to maintain appropriate levels of insulin and blood sugar. You'll note that I mentioned "net carbs." The Carb Manager software will compute the net carbs for you, so don't worry. However, it's critical to understand that total and net carbohydrates differ from one another. Your total carbohydrate intake less fiber equals your net carbohydrates. I want you to consume a lot of fiber because it helps break down dangerous estrogens. Your blood sugar should fall into the normal range of 70 to 90 when you keep your net carbohydrates under 50. Your body ought to be alerted to start producing ketones when you go into this range. The presence of ketones indicates that your liver has switched from burning carbohydrates to burning fat for energy. This is lovely. Weight reduction will happen more quickly after you train your body to make that change.

Your brain, particularly the pituitary and hypothalamus, which coordinate all hormone synthesis, are greatly benefited by ketones. There is a setting on your blood glucose monitor for ketones. Your ketone result should be greater than 0.5. We refer to that as nutritional ketosis, and the desired range is between 0.5 and 5.0. You are burning fat for energy as long as you are in that area.

I want to highlight a crucial aspect of decreasing your carbohydrate load before I go on to protein. It will be tempting to continue reducing your carb intake once you realize how efficiently your body operates in this low-carb environment. Frequently, this entails giving up veggies. This is not a good idea for a woman who is menopausal. Vegetables are necessary to break down estrogen. I have a comprehensive plan for you to feed the bacteria in your gut that breaks down estrogen, as you will see in the chapters that follow. Low keto diets for menopausal women are not something I support. In low-keto diets, limiting carbs to 20 grams is common. I recommend a ketogenic diet instead. By maintaining a ketogenic diet, you can consume plenty of greens and foods high in probiotics and prebiotics, which help break down estrogen. Net carbs should be kept at around 50 grams.

Protein

I want you to consider two factors when it comes to protein. The protein's quality comes first. Meat has the potential to be the most harmful food you consume. The animals we consume are typically fed a high-grain diet and frequently given growth hormones and antibiotic injections. You ingest whatever is put into that meat. These substances can mess with your hormones. Eating a healthy diet is the first step in getting enough protein. This means that you should prefer grass-fed, organic meats whenever possible. I refer to this as clean meat. Start looking at the ingredients in your meat and reading the labels. As time goes on, you'll begin to notice that many meat labels include the words "Raised without antibiotics," "Grass-fed," or "Hormone-free."

Let's look at how much protein you consume once you decide to eat only clean proteins. When someone adopts a low-carb diet, they frequently raise their protein intake. Since protein can also induce an increase in insulin levels, this is not a worthwhile trade-off. It's better to limit your daily protein intake to under 50 grams. Just make sure to enter your protein as well if you are using Carb Manager to calculate your net carbohydrates. This kind of measurement can be really helpful when you are first attempting to understand what your macro loads are.

Fat

Fat is the third macro I want you to start tracking. We have good and bad fat, much like protein. You must eat well and stay away from harmful foods to go through menopause. This is why. There are a trillion cells in your body. These cells have receptors on the outside that take hormones and let them into the cells to activate them. You'll feel wonderful after a hormone is able to enter the cell and perform its function. Toxins and poor fats are two things that can easily block these receptor sites. For a woman going through menopause, a blocked receptor site is the kiss of death. Your menopause symptoms will worsen if the hormone you are producing can't enter the cell because a receptor site is blocked. After all, you are already producing fewer hormones than ever before. Making sure you are eating healthy fats rather than unhealthy fats is the first step in keeping track of your fat macronutrients.

Common healthy fats include:

Olive oil

Avocado oil

Coconut oil

Grass-fed butter

Raw nuts and nut butter

Ghee

Fats you want to avoid are:

Canola oil

Vegetable oil

Partially hydrogenated oils

Soybean oil

Margarine

Corn oil

Safflower oil

Sunflower oil

Fats should be organic and not rancid, which is another crucial idea to keep in mind. Pesticides have the potential to jam up those hormone receptor sites. Pesticides are abundant in nonorganic lipids. By deciding to consume solely organic fats, you forego the pesticide dosage. If fats are old, they can also become rancid. Fats that have gone rancid will irritate the cell membrane and make it difficult for hormones to enter as well. To avoid having our oils become rancid, we use smaller bottles and replenish them more frequently in my home. If your oils smell rancid, you can usually determine quite quickly if they are. An oil that has gone bad has a distinct scent like damp cardboard.

The next stage is to examine how much fat you consume once you have cleaned up your fats. Revisit your Carb Manager once again. Make sure that more than 60% of the total amount of food you bring in each day is made up of fat. When it comes to fat, I advise against counting grams but rather percentages.

I realize this is unclear, but the key to managing your fat intake is to make sure that more than 60% of your daily calories come from good fats. In addition to healing your brain, reducing hunger, and providing you with pleasant, constant energy all day long, good fat also nourishes your cells. The secret to regulating your hormones and losing weight is in lowering your carbohydrate load, managing your protein, and increasing your fat. I know for many of you, the thought of eating that much fat is frightening, but I assure you it works. I have often witnessed this working for thousands of women.

If the information presented previously was unfamiliar to you, I want you to begin by becoming accustomed to these dietary modifications before you do anything further with your "meal. Before going on to the next phases, many of you will spend months in the aforementioned three steps (reduced carbs, moderate protein, higher fat). When I deal with a patient one-on-one, I make sure they adhere to these guidelines for at least 80% of the workweek. We move on to the following step, eating for your cycle, once they have established a routine of doing so.

Eat for your Cycle

You ought to have learned what I'm about to tell you when you first entered puberty. I don't understand why it isn't taught to all women that their nutritional needs vary depending on the stage of their cycle. You experience several hormonal surges during the month, and you can boost these hormones by consuming particular foods at particular points in your cycle.

It would be easy to skip this step because many of you either don't have a cycle or have an irregular one. Don't. Before we discuss how to adapt this for where you are in the menopause journey, let me first introduce you to the concept of eating for your cycle.

The follicular phase and the luteal phase were the two stages of ovulation that occurred while you were ovulating. The first to the fourteenth day of your cycle is the follicular phase. Your body is prepared to ovulate during this period when an egg will be released. The luteal phase is the second phase you experience each month. Your uterine lining prepares to receive a fertilized egg for implantation during this phase, which lasts from days fifteen to twenty-eight. The most crucial thing you need to know about these two phases right now is that you experience a significant hormone spike on days twelve to fourteen and days twenty-one to twenty-eight of every twenty-eight-day cycle. Your body needs the greatest progesterone during the second surge and the best estrogen during the first surge.

Estrogen and progesterone are rapidly decreasing as you enter the menopause years. Your periods are irregular because of this deterioration. Additionally, it's what's causing some of your symptoms. You may boost the development of both estrogen and progesterone by eating specific foods at specific times of the month once you are aware of this. Stay with me here, please. I see that this can be challenging, but I'll make it easier for you. The first thing to understand is which meals raise progesterone and estrogen levels. Some of my favorites are listed here:

Foods that increase estrogen:

Flax seeds

Sesame seeds

Soybeans/Edamame

Garlic

Dried apricots, dates, prunes

Peaches

Berries

Cruciferous foods like broccoli, cauliflower, and Brussels sprouts

Foods that increase progesterone:

Beans

Potatoes

Squashes

Quinoa

Tropical fruits

Citrus fruits

You'll note that several of these items have a greater carbohydrate content at first sight. You might even be thinking to yourself, "How can I eat potatoes and tropical fruits while keeping my carbohydrate load under fifty grams?" Eating for your cycle can help with this. The three situations I observe with my patients who are going through menopause are listed below. You will most likely fall into one of these three groups:

Maintain Your Regular Cycle

I want you to keep track of your cycle if you still have one. Now that I'm fifty, I'm following my period more faithfully than I did when I was a teenager. Now I make fun of myself. However I've discovered that eating for my period can significantly reduce the symptoms of menopause, so I've started keeping careful track of when my cycle comes and how much I eat to produce hormones.

I want you to pay attention to these two hormone surges after you get into the habit of monitoring your cycle. Your spike in estrogen is the first. Keep in mind that this normally occurs between days 12 and 14. I advise you to consume as many of the aforementioned

estrogen-building foods as you

can over these three days while avoiding counting macronutrients. Your progesterone surge occurs during the second surge. This surge normally starts around day twenty-one and lasts until you start bleeding. I want you to consume as many progesterone-stimulating foods as you choose at this period. You are not counting macros, just like on your estrogen-building days. Because this dietary pattern will have an impact on insulin, estrogen, and progesterone, I refer to it as a 28-Day Hormone Reset.

The questions of "Won't I gain weight?" and "Won't that throw me out of ketosis?" a common question I hear from the women I've taught this hormone-regulatory strategy. This is typically said by women who have succeeded greatly by taking the first steps I outlined in this chapter and who are afraid to make too many lifestyle changes since they feel so terrific.

If you share these worries, here's what I want you to do. You can still fast intermittently on these hormonally charged days. Make an effort to fast for at least fifteen hours throughout this period. I want you to be strict about adhering to the macros I specified at the beginning of this chapter and lean into some longer fasts like autophagy fasting or dinner-to-dinner fasting when you are not going through a hormone surge. Throw in several 36-hour fasts between days one and twelve, and fifteen to twenty-one for weight loss. This version will allow you to build hormones when your body requires them while also reaping the benefits of ketosis when your body is not attempting to produce these critical hormones.

Still not persuaded? Please understand that I am speaking from personal experience. I used to consume a few carbs and frequently go on long fasts when I first realized how amazing a low-keto and fasting lifestyle made me feel. This wrecked my sex hormones and exacerbated the symptoms of menopause. My period became erratic since my progesterone levels were so low. As my cycle progressed, I went from spotting to hemorrhaging so severe that I initially believed I should take the day off work to control my blood flow. The week before my period, I felt worried and incredibly irritable. When the anxiety would get high, I wouldn't even be able to unwind on the couch at home. These are all indications of dangerously low progesterone levels. The chaos ended as soon as I committed to the 28-day Hormone Reset regimen I outlined here. Everything stopped, including the worry as well as the spotting and bleeding. As I progress through menopause, I can already feel my cycles slowing down. However, it's a kinder and quieter ride. Now that I'm off the roller coaster, it feels more like my ovaries are gradually ceasing to function. Not like the erratic ups and downs I experienced a few years ago.

Have an Irregular Cycle

What should you do if you are uncertain of the timing of your cycle? The more you approach postmenopause, the more frequently this occurs.

When your cycle does arrive, start tracking it right away, is my first bit of advice. even if you have a day of bleeding. Make the first day of your cycle that. Afterward, adhere to the 28-Day Hormone Reset. The

28-Day Hormone Reset can help many of my patients, who have irregular cycles as a result of menopause, restore some regularity to their cycles. Keep in mind that between the ages of fifty-two and fifty-five is the typical age at which menopause is over. Menopause occurring before the age of fifty may indicate a physical imbalance that needs to be corrected. Your cycles will become regular again after using the above approach, which frequently corrects these imbalances.

What should you do if it is day 28 and you are still not experiencing symptoms of your period? If this applies to you, I want you to act as if day 29 is your first day even though you haven't had your period yet. then start at the beginning of the 28-day Hormone Reset. Continue this 28-day Hormone Reset if your period doesn't appear until you reach postmenopause status. If your period does appear at any point throughout this reset, simply restart day one when you first notice blood and continue with the 28-day Hormone Reset. Up until postmenopause, keep up this habit.

Have no cycle

What should you do if you are postmenopausal or are unsure of your menopausal status but haven't had a period in years? If you are under the age of fifty, I recommend that you complete the 28-Day Hormone Reset that I outlined above for the lady with an unpredictable cycle. Remember that you may have entered menopause prematurely. Many of the ladies in my practice who lost their cycle before the age of fifty will resume their periods after completing the 28-Day Hormone Reset. This is because you are regulating insulin and sex hormones with this eating style.

If you are over the age of fifty and haven't had a period in over a year, you are most likely postmenopausal. Because your ovaries are no longer functioning, the hormone-building days are less important for you. However, you still require estrogen and progesterone.   Some hormone-building days will be beneficial to you. You will also benefit from a more ketotic diet and will be able to conduct lengthier fasts anytime you choose. You don't need to consider timing, but you should keep hormones in mind. What I recommend is that you eat keto biotically for 80 percent of the time (fifty grams net carbs, fifty grams protein, and more than 60 percent fat) and eat hormone-building foods for the other 20 percent of the time (without counting macros). This might look like one or two days a week of hormone-building and the rest of the week xenobiotic. Confused? I understand that for some of you, this is a novel approach to food. I've summarized it below. Make sure to complete the instructions in the correct order. It will be tough to transition to eating for your cycle before you have mastered the xenobiotic strategy. First and foremost, master xenobiotics. Then proceed to consume for the duration of your cycle. If you are unsure about when your cycle will begin or end, simply follow the 28-Day Hormone Reset. You can't go wrong with that diet because you'll still be decreasing insulin with xenobiotics and boosting estrogen and progesterone with hormone-building days. In case you're still confused, I've summarized the 28-day hormone reset for you at the end of this chapter.

Steps to Eating to Balance Hormones

Take out all refined carbs.

Maintain a carbohydrate load of less than fifty net carbohydrates.

Consume just clean protein.

Maintain a protein intake of fewer than fifty grams.

Eat good fat and avoid harmful fat.

Make sure that at least 60% of the fat in your diet is healthy.

Once you've accomplished these steps,

proceed to the Hormone Reset for 28 Days

Hormone Reset for 28 Days

Day 1–11: Ketobolic with your choice of fast.

Day 12–14: Estrogen-boosting meals combined with intermittent fasting.

Day 15–21: Ketobiotic with your choice of fast.

Day 21-28: Progesterone-boosting meals combined with intermittent fasting

The ketogenic diet has grown in popularity in recent years, but it has garnered some negative feedback, particularly from women. I strongly believe that menopausal women should approach the ketogenic diet differently. What I've outlined for you in this chapter is a lovely method to reap the benefits of adopting keto while also conserving your gut bacteria and balancing your hormones. This is the finest of both worlds.

Chapter 6

Detoxify the Body

We are living in the most toxic period in human history. about the last sixty years, about eighty-seven thousand new compounds have entered our environment. These chemicals have found their way into our food, water, and soil. They're on our furniture, in our cosmetics, and woven into the fabric of our clothes. Toxins are even present in the dental chair, our annual flu vaccine, and pharmaceuticals. Many of these toxins, known as carcinogens, are known to cause cancer, while others, known as neurotoxins, damage neurological tissue. These poisons accumulate in your body's tissues, causing damage to healthy tissue. Toxins are bioaccumulating at a higher rate than ever before, causing the human body to suffer. The menopausal woman suffers the most from this increasing toxic burden. Let me explain why. Toxins prefer to build up in nerve tissue and fat. Both of these make up your brain. As a result, the brain is especially sensitive to toxic bioaccumulation. But keep in mind that you were miraculously created. You were born with a protective layer around your brain to keep hazardous chemicals out. It's known as the blood-brain barrier. It guards your brain except for three areas: the hypothalamus, pituitary, and pineal gland. These are the regions that regulate all hormone production. Toxins will disrupt your entire hormonal system once they settle here.

No matter how healthy your lifestyle is, detoxifying your brain is essential. It's a road back to rebalancing your already depleted hormones. This is precisely what occurred to me. When menopause hit me hard, I tried to live as clean and healthy a life as I could. But I still had enormous heat flashes, difficulties sleeping, mood swings, mental clarity issues, and low energy. My toxic load was the one thing I didn't handle. It wasn't until I learned how to detox these environmental toxins from my body that I was able to reclaim my life. In this chapter, I'll show you what toxins to search for and how to effectively detox them out of your body. The first thing to think about when it comes to detoxification is "Which toxins are affecting me the most?" in addition to "How am I going to get rid of them?" The hardest part of controlling your toxic load is realizing how many chemicals you are exposed to daily. I've tried to comprehend the over 87 thousand chemicals that have been introduced into our environment over the last fifty years. It has led me down rabbit holes of research in an attempt to determine which poisons are the most dangerous and which should be avoided. Rather than bore you with endless lists of compounds, I have divided them into three key categories: chemicals that last forever, endocrine disruptors, and heavy metals

Chemicals That Last Forever

PFA, which stands for super- and poly-fluoroalkyl, is the most prevalent everlasting chemical. This is a classification of over 5,000 chemicals that are extremely persistent in our environment and can quickly accumulate in our bodies. PFAs have been associated with immune system dysfunction, thyroid disorders, renal illness, increased cholesterol, and reproductive issues. The scariest aspect of these compounds is that they are classified as a probable carcinogen and will not quickly leave your body. According to research, these PFAs have a half-life of 92 years in our environment and eight years in the human body.

Can you see why they're termed "chemicals that last Forever "? These noxious substances intend to linger for a long time.

PFAs don't only influence one portion of your body; they can have a systemic effect as well. According to the Environmental Working Group, the immune system is particularly vulnerable to persistent chemicals, and new research indicates a strong link between PFA exposure and suppressed immune function, lower vaccine effectiveness, hypersensitivity, and an increased risk of autoimmune diseases.

Consider this for a minute. Have you ever been at work when there is a nasty cold going around? Some people get the flu while others do not. Why is this the case? What if your toxic load influences how robust your immune response is? What about the increase in autoimmune diseases? Genetics contribute to only 30% of all autoimmune diseases, according to new research. Toxins in the environment cause 70% of autoimmune diseases. Women are more likely than men to have autoimmune disorders, and 85 percent or more of individuals with multiple autoimmune diseases are female. These autoimmune disorders frequently manifest during times of significant hormonal shifts, such as menopause.

How do you stay away from these chemicals? Unfortunately, it is practically hard to avoid them entirely.

They can be found in your drinking water, food packaging, furniture, mattresses, carpet treatments, Teflon cookware, and even your clothing.

You can decrease your exposure by taking a few wise precautions. Here are a few examples:

Replace your Teflon pans with cast iron pans.

Prepackaged items in Styrofoam or cardboard to-go containers should be avoided.

Look for organic materials while selecting furniture.

Purchase a reverse osmosis water filter.

Disruptors of the Endocrine System

Endocrine-disrupting chemicals (EDCs) are very common in our surroundings. You may have heard about endocrine disruptors concerning hormonal cancers such as breast or ovarian cancer. However, these substances do not have to cause cancer to cause difficulties. They can upset your estrogen and progesterone balance, causing hair loss, hot flashes, anxiety, insomnia, and weight gain for no apparent cause. The following are the most common endocrine disruptors:

Bisphenol A (BPA) plastics

Polychlorinated biphenyls (PCBs)

Dichlorodiphenyltrichloroethane (DDT)

Dioxins

Pesticides

Parabens

Phthalates

Heavy metals

Endocrine disruptive substances are known to inhibit hormone receptor sites. Remember how the brain instructs particular endocrine glands to secrete hormones? Even though your brain is healthy and your endocrine glands are operating well, you may still show signs of hormonal imbalance owing to blocked receptor sites. This is a common occurrence while dealing with thyroid issues.

Many women have thyroid symptoms, but their doctors will

look at their blood work and say they are fine. So why don't they feel better? Worse, many women are prescribed thyroid medication yet still feel terrible. If this describes you, your thyroid problems are most likely caused by blocked receptor sites rather than a gland disease.

Reduced exposure to endocrine disruptors will make a significant difference in your hormonal health. The following are the most significant steps you can take to reduce your EDCs.

1. Consume Organic

Organic food is no longer only for hippies. It is intended for everybody who wishes to keep healthy and avoid disease. Pesticides are not only known carcinogens, but they also disrupt hormone receptor sites. Receptor sites are holes in cells that allow hormones to enter and activate a specific activity in your body. T3 hormone, for example, enters cells and triggers metabolism. If a poison obstructs a receptor site, the hormone cannot enter, resulting in a delayed metabolism. Your thyroid gland is an endocrine gland that is particularly prone to pesticides. Pesticides can obstruct thyroid hormone receptor sites and kill healthy thyroid tissue. The thyroid gland is often referred to as the "canary in the coal mine." When your thyroid gland malfunctions, it indicates that your toxic burden is high.

Organic foods are now widely available. If money is an issue, the first place to look is at your meat. Pesticides are found in higher concentrations in animals than in fruits and vegetables.

2. Throw away the plastic

BPA plastics are also wreaking havoc on your hormones. They not only harm all of your endocrine glands, but they also block receptor sites and settle in your brain. If you still use plastic bags or containers for your food, it is time to quit. Plastics leak into your meals and contribute to menopausal symptoms.

In my house, we utilize glass containers to store leftovers as well as all of our water bottles. This was a simple change that took only one day of walking through the kitchen and throwing out anything that resembled plastics. It's a worthwhile endeavor that will spare you a lot of sleepless nights and hot flashes.

3. Develop your toxic lense

I'd like you to begin viewing everything you eat, drink, breathe, or touch through a hazardous lens. Are there chemicals in here? you might wonder. Is there a natural version of this? These are referred to as lateral alterations. You're simply replacing a harmful version with a natural one. Air fresheners are an excellent example of a little lateral modification that can have a significant impact on your hormones. Car and home air fresheners are proven endocrine disruptors. Can essential oils and diffusers be used in their place? What about packaged foods? "What can you create for yourself?"

When you begin to view things through a toxic lens, it will become second nature to select the healthier, nontoxic options. The first stage is to become aware. It's like going vehicle shopping. When you know the car you want, you can find it anywhere on the road. Toxins will behave similarly. You will not only begin to recognize dangerous goods, but you will also acquire taste buds that will inform you whether a food is fresh or toxic. I assure you that it is a muscle that can be developed. Your long-term health will considerably improve after you train it.

heavy metals

A menopausal woman's worst nightmare is heavy metals. Many metals, such as lead and mercury, reside in your tissues and are released into your bloodstream during hormonal changes such as puberty, pregnancy, and menopause. Once in the bloodstream, they frequently travel to the brain, where they disrupt the regions of your brain that regulate your hormones.

Heavy metals are the most dangerous of all poisons. They may be the primary cause of your memory loss, feelings of depression and irritability, and inability to sleep. Many of these metals were gathered inadvertently by you years ago. In certain situations, your mother passed on your large mental burden to you while you were still in the womb.

Some of you have a high mental load as a result of generational exposure from your mother or grandmother. This was certainly true during my menopausal experience.

Because heavy metals are released from stored tissues, they might creep up on you. When a menopausal woman says, "Out of nowhere, I started having trouble sleeping," or "All my old tricks for losing weight are no longer working," or "I feel sorry for my poor husband because I am just so irritable and easily agitated," I know she is suffering from heavy metal toxicity. Those are classic symptoms of metal release.

Lead and mercury are two of the most frequent elements that can contribute to your menopausal roller coaster.

Lead

I've tested thousands of my patients for heavy metals, and not one has come back lead-free. Lead is ingrained in your bones. It is secreted into your bloodstream during menopause, aggravating nerves, weakening bones, and decreasing your memory. I can't tell you how many examples I've encountered of menopausal women with high lead levels who are osteoporotic, despondent, and struggling to recover their words. These are typical symptoms of lead toxicity. Lead strikes me as a suppressor. It slows down your thoughts, steals your joy, weakens your bones, and leaves you in dull chronic discomfort.

Mercury

Mercury, on the other hand, is stimulating. It is the metal that causes agitation, irritability, and restlessness, as well as keeping you up at night. It acts more as a stimulant. Menopausal women already have high levels of anxiety owing to dropping progesterone levels, but add a high mercury burden to that and you've got one grumpy menopausal woman.

There are steps you may take to reduce your exposure to dangerous heavy metals. Heavy metals are most commonly found in the following locations:

Dentist (Amalgam fillings and crowns)

Influenza vaccinations

Fish

Renovating an ancient house with lead paint

Cosmetics, particularly lipstick

Dishware made of ceramic

consuming water

Vegetables and fruit are cultivated on heavy metal-contaminated soil.

You can get rid of these toxins before you lose hope. However, detoxifying from environmental poisons requires a different approach. Fasting, autophagy stimulation, juice cleaning, or colon cleansing will not help. When detoxing heavy metals and environmental pollutants, I prescribe four specific steps.

1. Understand your toxic load

Toxins live in stored tissues, so it's difficult to assess how toxic your body is. Blood and hair tests will only reveal what is currently in your system. They will not reveal what is contained in bone, fat, or nerve tissue. This is why we offer a triggered heavy metal test to our patients. This is a urine test in which a stimulating agent, such as DMSA, is used to draw metals from stored tissues and transport them to your urine for measurement.

Testing your hazardous load might assist you in developing a plan of action. Without this strategy, you may never know how much and for how long you need to detox.

2. Make your detox pathways more accessible.

Keep in mind that you are dealing with man-made synthetic compounds. Before beginning any form of thorough detox, make sure your detoxification organs are healthy and ready for the work. Your liver, intestine, kidneys, skin, and lymph system are the key detoxification organs.

When it comes to facilitating the detoxification process and supporting these organs in my patients, some of the techniques I have discovered to be most effective include:

Dry Brushing: Dry brushing is a method that involves using an organic, natural brush on your skin. Enhancing blood circulation and encouraging lymph flow and evacuation, aids in detoxification. During the exfoliation process, dry brushing can clear clogged pores. Additionally, it stimulates your nervous system, which may leave you feeling energized. I adore using a dry brush.

Infrared saunas: Infrared saunas are distinct from the typical saunas used in gyms. Your cells become heated from the inside out by infrared. It is very similar to how a fever develops. The ability to burn off infections, expel poisons, and restore cellular respiration are all possible when cells heat up from the inside out.

Coffee Enemas: As frightening as a coffee enema may sound, so many of my patients report that it has changed their lives. Enemas of coffee are just what they sound like. You use coffee as an enema in place of water. When coffee is ingested in this way, it widens the common bile duct, which is the liver's channel for excreting toxins.

Red light therapy: Healing red light. In my clinic, red light is frequently used to encourage cellular repair. Red light heals the outer cell membrane and activates your mitochondria when it enters a cell. The component of the cell that starts detoxification within the cell is the mitochondria.

PEMF: Visualize your mitochondria as the cellular battery. Your cells will continue to be irritated and unable to expel toxins if your battery is low. Healthy electromagnetic frequencies called PEMF are sent to the cells, energizing the mitochondria and allowing them to detoxify once more.

Hyperbaric Oxygen Chambers: As you detox, oxygen is also beneficial to your cells. Our cells' capacity to take in oxygen is impaired as we become older. Compressed oxygen, or hyperbaric oxygen, makes it simple for oxygen to enter cells. The mitochondria will recover when your cells get more oxygen, which will make it easier for them to push poisons out of the cells.

Supplements: Do you recall methylation? Well, for methylation to take place within the cells, numerous nutrients are required. nutrients including

CoQ10 and B vitamins. We take a supplement called MORS by Systemic Formulas when we are helping a patient to open up their detox pathways. This vitamin promotes healthy methylation and aids in cell detoxification.

3. Get rid of any toxins from your body.

I guarantee that once you understand how toxins affect your menopause symptoms, you'll be driven to start a brain detox as soon as possible. Everyone wants the toxins to leave their brains as soon as possible. I understand. Your menopause symptoms will significantly alter if your brain is free of poisons.

Keep in mind that toxins will pass through your liver, intestines, kidneys, and lymph system as they are eliminated from your brain. You should cleanse those organs first, in my opinion. If not, it would be equivalent to attempting to empty your full kitchen trash can into your overflowing curbside garbage can.

The toxins will simply leak into further tissues.

Following are some methods I've discovered to be effective for cleansing the body:

Glutathione levels can be raised by taking supplements or eating more cruciferous vegetables.

By boosting healthy fats, cellular membrane performance is improved.

Utilize binders such as DMSA, zeolites, or activated charcoal.

Enhance methylation by taking supplements or eating more foods high in sulfur.

4. Get rid of brain toxins

You regain control of your life at this point. You begin to feel more like yourself at this point. I enjoy brain detoxing because it makes me feel as though a magic wand has been waved over my mind. I've done so many brain detoxes by this point that whenever I start one, my brain returns to feeling ecstatic, clear, and focused. I found the following techniques useful for brain detoxification:

Boost the synthesis of ketone

Keep in mind that while you fast, you naturally produce ketones. Fasting for lengthier periods to promote ketone generation can be beneficial if you're detoxing your brain.

Massive mineral intake

To function normally, your brain needs certain minerals. A person can experience severe depression from a simple zinc deficiency. Because toxins frequently occupy mineral receptor sites, your brain will require more minerals to function normally when you remove the toxins. When you are on a brain detox, I strongly advise you to up your mineral intake. The mineral supplement we suggest is made by Systemic Formulas and is branded as MIN.

Add an alpha lipoic acid supplement, such as Brain DTX

Getting across the blood-brain barrier is one of the difficulties we face while trying to cleanse the brain. Very few nutrients can get past this formidable barrier. We advise taking a product called Brain DTX to detox your brain. It contains a nutrient called alpha lipoic acid, which can go deep inside your brain and shake toxins free.

Add binders like DMSA and Zeolites, which are found in Cytodetox, to your diet.

The use of binders is the secret to all detoxification. Toxins will be bound as they leave the cells. This is crucial to prevent the reabsorption of poisons. Our preferred binder for brain detoxification is Cytodetox because it has the greatest capacity to magnetize metals.

Weekly usage of hyperbaric oxygen chambers

Driving oxygen into the brain cells as poisons leave them can be therapeutic. In our clinic, we advise patients to undergo brain detoxification in hyperbaric oxygen chambers.

Weekly chiropractic adjustments

Chiropractic may be well-known for treating back and neck pain, but a recent study demonstrates that it is capable of much more. We now understand that a chiropractic adjustment enhances the flow of cerebrospinal fluid into and out of the brain. The process of detoxification is carried out by the cerebral spinal fluid. A chiropractic adjustment also shifts the brain's focus from the fight-or-flight response to one of possibilities and hope. Our patients who include weekly chiropractic adjustments in their brain detoxes recover more quickly and experience fewer withdrawal symptoms.

When I talk about toxins, I always feel depressed. I am aware that understanding and getting rid of these poisons from your body is a difficult undertaking. I made an effort to address my menopausal roller coaster solely through dietary modifications. It was a failure. I felt like myself again after learning about toxins and making the commitment to frequently detoxifying. I see that many more women would experience the same thing. The detox offers relief from difficult menopause symptoms. Your hormones can be balanced again, and you'll feel more like yourself as a result.

Steps to Continue Detoxing Your Life

1. Ensure that you eat organic food whenever possible.

2. Discard the plastic.

3. Develop a poisonous lens

4. Recognise your harmful load

5. Let your detox pathways work.

6. Remove toxins from your system.

7. Remove toxins from your head.

I have devoted countless hours to learning and using various forms of natural healing on the human body. Few things in a person's life have been as amazing as detoxifying. We are in such a toxic era, and our Toxic buckets are quickly overflowing. Detoxing correctly can save your life.

An excess of pollutants is the cause of the health issues that plague so many individuals. When your cells are full of poisons, they cannot repair themselves. It's time to detox if you've tried everything to heal yourself yet feel like nothing is working. I can assure you that when you get rid of these poisons from your body, miracles take place. You'll recover quicker, feel better, and be able to perform at a higher level of health than you could have ever imagined possible.

Chapter 7

Stay Forever Young

I consider everything I've taught you so far to be lifestyle hacking. Applying these concepts will enable you to improve your health to a degree you might not have thought possible and help you thrive throughout your menopause journey.

I want to introduce you to a term right now that is popular in the anti-aging community. It is known as biohacking. Biohacks share three characteristics. They are safe, natural ways to achieve your goals, and they operate with your body's knowledge. Biohacking is a very fascinating field. It's challenging to keep up with the research on all of the new biohacking tools that are being developed every day. The fact that we will become less reliant on medications and surgery as more of these hacks are made accessible to the general population is maybe what excites people the most. This is so motivating!

Our current era is fascinating. More people than ever before want to slow down the aging process. Baby boomers do not want to get old as their parents did. The elderly suffering from dementia, Alzheimer's disease, and persistent arthritis at younger ages make Gen Xers think, "Not for me." Different ages are desired by people. As a result, a whole industry of biohacking has emerged.

We have some interesting new biohacking tools that are becoming accessible for the average person to employ to delay the aging process. technologies that have been the subject of extensive research. Some of these tools can be helpful to you as you go through the menopause years. Red light treatment, infrared saunas, hyperbaric oxygen chambers, PEMF, vibration therapy, and brain training are some of my favorites for menopausal women.

Before I outline any of these fascinating technologies, I want to caution you. Your way of life will either make or break you. Biohacking is not a substitute for a way of living that puts the hormonal hierarchy first. Even though it may be tempting to enter a hyperbaric oxygen chamber to treat your low mood and memory issues, you will still need to address any bad habits you may have in your daily routine. You will thrive during the menopause years thanks to the interaction between lifestyle hacks and biohack technologies.

In light of this, allow me to introduce you to some incredible hacks that will improve your hormones and slow down the aging process.

Red Light Treatment

You are exposed to a lot of blue light when you spend the entire day indoors, sitting in front of a computer with fluorescent lights blazing down on you. Certain blue lights can harm your cells and accelerate the aging process.

This is especially true in tissues like your skin that are exposed to blue light frequently.

However, not all light is harmful. Your cells can be revitalized and made to live longer by healing lights. One of the lights is the red light. Red light is emitted naturally at sunrise and sunset. But if you're like most people, you don't frequently run outside to catch this light. Red light therapy is helpful in this situation.

Even 10 minutes a day of red light exposure to various parts of your body can have a significant impact on your hormones and collagen formation, possibly even reducing joint inflammation. There are several excellent red lights available.

There is extensive research on this therapeutic red light. Collagen skin regeneration may be the most exciting option for postmenopausal women. Red light therapy has been shown in numerous trials to reduce the appearance of aging in the skin. Red and near-infrared light have both been demonstrated to increase collagen, reduce wrinkles, and improve skin tone for a more youthful appearance. Our endocrine glands are known to respond to red light therapy. in particular, your thyroid.

Infrared sauna

Detoxification, weight loss, and skin renewal are all possible with infrared saunas. Your toxic burden may become apparent when you go through menopause. You may acquire weight more quickly as a result of this. For removing those toxins organically, infrared saunas are a fantastic tool.

Infrared is like a fever, in your mind. Cells get heated inside as a result. These toxins may be held in the cells, but the heat induces them to release them. Don't forget about the toxin-induced receptor site blockade. Unblocking those receptor sites and reactivating your hormones can be accomplished with the use of infrared saunas. The skin can be repaired with infrared saunas. Because only 80% to 85% of the sweat produced in a far infrared sauna is water and the remaining portion contains toxic heavy metals, cholesterol, fat-soluble toxins, sodium, ammonia, and uric acid, far infrared saunas are thought to be more effective than traditional saunas at moving toxins through the skin.

(HBOT) Hyperbaric Oxygen Chamber

Your cells become oxygen-saturated as you age. Even with exercises like high-intensity training, it becomes challenging for you to drive additional oxygen into your body. Yet we require oxygen. It benefits the mitochondria in your cells, which make ATP to provide you with energy. Compressing oxygen is the only method to get it into these aging cells. similar to adding carbonation to a bottle. An oxygen chamber is used to do that. Your cells can be penetrated by compressed oxygen, which has a healing effect.

Although hyperbaric oxygen is frequently utilized for muscle recovery and athletic performance, it is also having a significant impact on brain health. More oxygen is needed for the brain than any other organ in the body. It is miraculous when someone with repeated brain injuries or memory loss is placed in an oxygen chamber. Oxygen helps the brain to recover. Impressive study has also been done on hyperbaric oxygen. Treatments with hyperbaric oxygen have been shown to promote angiogenesis, which results in the growth of new blood vessels in tissue, and to prompt the release of stem cells from our bone marrow into the bloodstream. It has also been demonstrated that hyperbaric oxygen chambers can reduce inflammation.

PEMF

Do you know how your cell phone loses its battery and needs to be recharged? The cells in our bodies experience the same things, according to recent research. However, it takes years for it to happen instead of a few days. Although we refer to it as aging or feel like we are just slowing down, your body's cells are designed to keep you healthy for well over a hundred years. At fifty, they are not supposed to start to slow down.

Your cells have a variety of needs, and electromagnetic energy is one of them. The earth provides us with electromagnetic energy. Have you ever observed that after being in nature, you feel more at ease and peaceful? That's because you received a healthy dose of the electromagnetic energy from the ground, which charged your cells.

In the modern environment, poisons, poor nutrition, inflammatory lipids, blue lights from cell phones, and harmful EMFs from Wi-Fi that roar through our homes and offices all target our cells. These harm our cells and sap their strength.

Where PEMF can be useful is in this situation. Our cells can be recharged by pulsed electromagnetic frequencies, which are also beneficial to them. PEMF is, in my opinion, the body's version of my phone charger. Your cells are getting refilled when you sit in a PEMF chair. The body can heal from chronic pain, chronic exhaustion, and even depression with the help of this additional power, which is proving to help provide the body with the vitality it needs.

Vibration Therapy

Have you ever observed that as you get older, keeping your muscles requires more effort? Well, let me introduce vibration treatment to you. It's a fantastic tool for a woman going through the menopause. You most likely already have vibration therapy at your gym without even realizing it.

My love for vibration therapy stems from two factors. The first is that compared to simply standing on level ground, standing on a vibration plate requires the engagement of hundreds more muscles. Because of this, fitness instructors adore it. On a vibration plate, performing a "squat forces more muscles to function with less effort from the user. In my workplace, vibration plates are frequently used to strengthen people's postural muscles and prevent the rounded forward head position that comes with aging or prolonged cell phone use.

The fact that this therapy makes your bones stronger is the second reason I adore it. This is beneficial to menopausal women. Your bones are encouraged to retain calcium and phosphorus by vibration therapy. Your overall profile of bone density may be improved by this. Additionally, it has been demonstrated that whole-body vibration raises the levels of growth hormone and testosterone in postmenopausal women's serum, preventing sarcopenia and osteoporosis.

Conclusion

Glad you finally reached the conclusion. In this book, I intend to take you on a journey that inspires you and restores your faith in humanity. I wish you could be where I am and witness the thousands of women who reset their menopause symptoms every day by following the five steps I laid down for you. Keep in mind that every chapter contains a different level of healing for you.

Reread the chapters you believe require the most improvement by going back and doing so. Reread the Chapters where I taught you about the hormonal hierarchy and which hormones are affecting your symptoms if you get off track on your menopause journey. Reread those chapters if you are having issues with your weight, energy, hot flashes, or mental clarity, then start establishing a fasting and keto-biotic lifestyle for yourself.

Want to sleep but can't? Do you have hair loss? Do you feel as though your memory isn't what it once was? Then go back and get acquainted with the pollutants in your environment that could be disrupting your hormone balance.

Never lose sight of the fact that your magnificent body was born with a built-in healing mechanism as you go through this process. Contrary to what you have been taught, your body is far stronger. I understand that the difficulties you've faced do not seem remarkable, but I assure you that there is a tremendous chance for healing during this difficult menopause journey.

A mirror is menopause. Your body is giving you gifts that it wants you to address, such as the symptoms that are there in front of you. My sincerest wish for you is that you embrace rather than demonize these symptoms. They take place for you; they do not take place for you.

Concerning the state of our planet right now, my heart bleeds.

However, no one is more at risk than a woman who is going through menopause. Hormones offer a defense. As you enter your postmenopausal years and lose that protection, you become more vulnerable to many illnesses. Postmenopausal women are more likely to have osteoporosis, hormonal malignancies, cardiovascular disease, arthritis, dementia, Alzheimer's, and diabetes. You have a chance as you wait for the peri-to-post-menopause transition to end. The trajectory of your health is something you can change. You may regain control by making the lifestyle modifications I've described here. Chronic illness does not develop suddenly. Cancer cells form over many years of living poorly. Illness stops spreading when you pay attention to your body's demands.

Your body wants to heal, regardless of the diagnosis that has been given to you, the number of toxins you have been exposed to, or the number of doctors who have given you a dismal prognosis. It is prepared for this time. It wants to collaborate rather than compete with you. You possess a strong intelligence that is aware of what to do. You will discover just how powerful your body was designed to be when you put the methods I outlined in this book into practice.

You already have what you need to thrive during the menopause years. Return to these book's pages if you sense that you are veering off course. Review the chapters in which your hormones are discussed. Remember the hormonal hierarchy and the fact that balancing estrogen, progesterone, and testosterone is more successful when cortisol and insulin are in balance. Return to the steps that make up the Menopause cure if you get off track and sense that your symptoms have control over you. Take these measures as a road map to help you get out of this situation.